THE IMMUNE SYSTEM:

A NUTRITIONAL APPROACH

by
Louise Tenney

The information contained in this book is in no way to be considered as prescription for any ailment. The prescription of any medication should be made by a duly licensed physician.

Published by:
Woodland Health Books

Printed in U.S.A.

REFERENCES

Immerman, Alan. "Intestinal Bacteria," <u>Vegetarian Times</u>, January/February 1980.

The Rodale Report. "Eight Ways to Strengthen Your Immune System," February 1984.

Tenney, Louise. "Immune System Do's and Don'ts."
Today's Healthy Eating
Today's Herbal Health

THE IMMUNE SYSTEM:

A NUTRITIONAL APPROACH

by
Louise Tenney

INTRODUCTION: MARK'S IMMUNE SYSTEM

Mark was born with a weak immune system. In Iridology it is known as "weak constitution." This weakness determined his general health pattern after he was born. He inherited poor health, low vitality and toxins from his parents. The mother's improper diet during pregnancy set the stage for this condition. Even the diets of grand-parents and ancestors played a role.

Mark's poor immune system manifested itself when he was only three months old. He developed an ear infection and was subsequently given antibiotics. This pattern continued for the first three years of his life. Mark would get any virus or disease that floated by. Sudden fevers with attendant convulsions were a periodic occurrence during his first five years. Phenobarbital was the medication prescribed for the convulsions. The doctors told Mark's parents that he would have to be on this medication for his entire life, with other drugs as well. Mark endured a battery of tests, including brain scan tests. The medical profession could not find any abnormalities in the brain waves. However, they still insisted he be given this drug continually. When he was five years old it was recommended that he take it <u>daily,</u> but the parents decided to discontinue it altogether. Mark never had another convulsion after his fifth birthday! Taking him off the medication seemed to be the answer to his problem.

Mark was a very cheerful, active child, and this was in his favor. Other children gravitated to him because of his pleasant disposition. However, his childhood was fraught with battling sickness. He caught all kinds of diseases. When he was 1-1/2 years old he became ill with Roseola Infantum. This is a non-infectious viral infection, characterized by a high fever and rash. He was rushed to the isolation unit of the hospital, but when he broke out with the rash the doctors realized what it was.

Mark had a bout with walking pneumonia, pleurisy and strep throat. During his teen years he fought colds, flu and infections. Once, when playing racquetball, he developed a blister and the next day had blood poisoning! His body just could not withstand any type of adverse condition, because of his lack of antibodies.

At the age of 21 he caught undulant fever. This was a result of drinking raw milk while living abroad. His symptoms were numerous. He was afflicted with chills, fever, severe headache, muscular aches and pains, loss of weight, joint pain, backache, weakness, nervous irritability, insomnia, sweating, and mental depression. This was the turning point in his life. He decided to try herbs, vitamins, and minerals. He drank Pau d'Arco tea by the quarts and took acidophilus, garlic, calcium, and vitamins A and C. Protein drinks were consumed for their amino acids, and he took B-complex tablets. Mark was given an herbal lower bowel formula with Cascara Sagrada to keep his bowels open. Also, an herbal blood purifier to clean his blood was taken. This nutritional regime enabled him to successfully conquer the undulant fever within three months.

When he was in Hawaii and 22 years old, Mark stepped on a piece of coral. Although the scratch was superficial, it became infected, then developed into a severe case of blood poisoning. He didn't have his herbs with him and was forced to rely on staph medications and antibiotics. When he was 24, he and his wife baby-sat her nephews, who had chickenpox. Two weeks later he came down with them!

Mark is now 25 years old. He knows that he has to take care of his health. If he doesn't eat right he pays the price with colds, flu, or whatever is going around. He must avoid red meat, milk, and sweet products. His immune system needs to be vitalized through comprehensive nutritional support.

THE IMMUNE SYSTEM: HOW IT WORKS

The key to prevention and treatment of diseases is a healthy, well-functioning immune system. This wonderful apparatus we were born with is not the source of protection it once was. The body can be weakened to the point that it does not respond to the normal intake of nutrients. The immune system can accumulate damage, becomes defective and consequently cannot do its job. This problem plays a role in most degenerative diseases. The immune system can become harmed in a short period of time if we abuse our bodies, to the extent it cannot repair itself. This is especially true if we do not supplement our bodies with vitamins, minerals and herbs. These concentrated foods help repair the damage inflicted by the accumulation of toxic materials.

The immune system is designed to be genetically-programmed to shelter you from disease. It *will* protect you, if you keep it in top shape. The immune system is equipped with glands, cells, organs, and proteins to fight off flus, colds, even cancer. With all of the diseases in the world ready to invade your body, your immune system must be prepared to battle these scourges.

The immune system has several responsibilities. One of them is to fight illness, another one is gathering information on the disease and reporting back to the various cells and organs, which are part of the immune network. Another part produces "ammunition" which will destroy the foreign invaders. The intricacy of the immune system keeps us safe from bacteria, viruses, yeast or fungal infections. Other toxins and organisms are kept at bay and cannot infiltrate our tissues or do damage when the immune system is functioning properly. The immune system, with its specific cells scattered throughout the body, has the unique power to recognize threats to survival. These threats are then ingested or devoured. They are first isolated, neutralized, then destroyed.

How kind are you to your immune system? Do you make it work twice as hard by eating devitalized, junk foods? The poor immune system has to then extract meager quantities of nutrients from these foods and limp along, disposing of the non-nutrients anywhere it can. They usually end up as an advertisement of the quality of our diet...as fat around the stomach, thighs, etc.

Low immunity can manifest itself as fatigue, irritability, and general susceptibility to disease and infections. Give your immune system a break! It is your friend and wants to help you! The key to a healthy immune system is proper intake of nutritious elements. The body can then distribute them in abundance and fortify the cells against the ravages of stress, pollution, and disease. Sometimes there are diseases so prevalent today, we think of them as "plagues."

3

MODERN DAY PLAGUES

There are several modern day plagues which affect the immune system. The following are major ones of which you should be aware:

Aids--A.I.D.S. (Acquired Immunity Deficiency Syndrome), is a disorder that alters the body's ability to protect itself. It is a complete breakdown of the immune system. When the immune system is functioning properly, the AIDS virus is destroyed by the white blood cells. This disease is now in epidemic proportions and is filtering into the mainstream of society. Years ago, almost all of those who contracted the illness were homosexuals, but small children and others are contracting it. Some of the ways are through blood transfusions, intravenous drug abuse, tattoo needles, and prostitution. This virus can be transmitted without showing any symptoms of the disease to those who carry it. Prevention is the only answer. The immune system is the most vital factor in preventing this disease.

Candida Albicans--A yeast invader, to weaken the immune system. It is in epidemic proportions. This disease can produce mild symptoms or create pain, fatigue, and mental anguish. This is created by the medical profession who so freely prescribed antibiotics. Doctors are now realizing that antibiotics should not be given freely but now they are given to animals in their feed, assuring a constant supply of them in our food.

Herpes--Herpes is another modern day plague. Herpes is commonly known as fever blisters, canker, or cold sores. It is a recurrent viral infection, (often in the same site). Herpes infection above the waist is called Herpes Simplex Type 1. Herpes infection below the waist is called Herpes Simplex Type II. Herpes is a virus, a parasite that feeds off the nutrients of other cells. This virus enters the body through the skin and sets up residence in the nerve at the base of the spine, deep inside the body. Recurrences are triggered by stress, fever, menstruation, lack of sleep, overwork, fatigue, inadequate nutrition, emotional upset, sexual intercourse, too much exposure to sun, wind and cold weather, and friction from wearing tight clothing.

Women who have active Herpes II may have an increased chance of miscarriage or premature delivery. More serious is the chance of infection of the newborn. Herpes II infection in infants can cause brain or neurological damage and blindness. Sixty percent of the newborns

4

who catch Herpes II die. Herpes in women has been linked to cancer of the cervix. It does not automatically lead to cancer, but if the immune system is weak, it is possible. An inefficient immune system is triggered by certain emotional or physical factors, along with poor nutrition.

Toxic Shock Syndrome--Toxic Shock Syndrome affects menstruating women in their late teens or early twenties. It afflicts those who use highly absorbent synthetic fiber tampons, which are thought to trigger Staphyloccus Aures. This organism produces the toxins which cause Toxic Shock Syndrome. It is felt that one cause could be the absorbing effect depleting the body of magnesium, which protects the immune system. Many women have been stricken by this disease quite suddenly. In 1985 it was reported over the news that 114 women had died from this disease. These women usually experienced nausea, diarrhea, and dizziness, accompanied by a sudden high fever. This was often followed by a rash, peeling skin, and possibly shock, unconsciousness, paralysis and even death. A sharp drop in blood pressure is another symptom of this syndrome. Recovery is often a long and painful process.

Reye's Syndrome--Reye's Syndrome is a childhood disease which targets children under 18. Parents have been warned not to give their children aspirin if they are suspected of having chicken pox or the flu. This combination seems to precipitate the syndrome. One group of children in Canada developed Reye's Syndrome after suffering from an influenza viral infection. This disease produces fever, vomiting, disturbance of consciousness progressing to coma and convulsions. It causes fatty infiltration of the liver and kidneys, with cerebral edema and many other destructive effects. A weakened immune system will promote susceptibility to this unfortunate problem.

Crib Death--Crib Death (Sudden Infant Death Syndrome) is the leading cause of death for American babies over a week old. Parents put an apparently healthy baby to bed at night and find it dead in the morning. Each year thousands of babies between four weeks and seven months of age die in their sleep. This is a very devastating experience that no parent should have to endure. Crib death may result from a breakdown in the babies' immune systems. Babies are born with naturally low immunity, but acquire a certain amount from their mothers' antibodies in the placenta. Breast fed infants are relatively healthier and suffer less mortality than the bottle-fed babies. SIDS is preponderately a disease which affects these artificially fed infants. Bottle-fed babies suffer from deficiencies in oxygen. This causes bacteria to become pathogenic, parasitic and virulent. Virulent bacteria produces viruses which exhaust vitamin C in the body. This causes a weakening in the immune system. A lack of other essential nutrients may be involved in this syndrome.

Legionnaires' Disease--This is another disease caused by a breakdown in the immune system. It occurs more often in persons who are middle-aged to elderly, who have lymphoma or other disorders. It receives its name from the peculiar, highly publicized illness that struck 182 people (29 of whom died), at an American Legion convention in Philadelphia the summer of 1976. It is an acute bronchopneumonia produced by a gram-negative bacillus. Again, the immune system plays a vital role in protecting one from this sickness.

Youth Suicide--Suicide is increasing rapidly in the United States, and is reaching epidemic proportions. The highest rate of suicide is among senior citizens, but the largest sudden numbers are among adolescents. Dr. Laurence Schwab (Let's Live Magazine, January 1984), says that the most appalling discovery among the youth suicides and those who tried to commit suicide was their rotten nutrition. Inadequate nutrition was the predominant factor found in the diets of most of them. The diets of these teenagers usually consist of junk food like caffeine drinks, numerous white sugar products, and no intake of food supplements. Alcohol and drug consumption is prevalent. It is well known that alcohol and drugs are the number one cause of malnutrition in the United States. Many authorities in nutrition regard low intake of proper nutrients as being especially damaging to the immune system.

STRENGTHENING THE IMMUNE SYSTEM

According to experts, there are eight ways to strengthen the immune system.

1. **Eat Properly.** "It's not that certain nutrients affect the immune system," says Purdue University nutrition professor, Thomas Petro, Ph.D. "It's that every nutrient affects the immune system."

Indeed, studies suggest that each of the major vitamins (A, B, C, D and E) plays a part in protecting you against unfriendly organisms. Zinc is vital for keeping the immune system healthy. Eat a well-balanced diet comprised of fresh fruits and vegetables, lean meat, nuts and seeds, beans and whole grain products, and low-fat dairy products to ensure a variety of nutrient intake.

2. **Exercise Often.** Exercise can stimulate immunity to disease. In one experiment, rats were found to be more disease-resistant after being injected with blood samples of people who had just exercised. Their body temperatures increased slightly, the white blood cells multiplied, and other changes were noted, showing evidence that their immune systems were ready to battle any unwelcome microbe.

3. **Avoid Stressful Situations.** Some stress is good because it can serve as a motivator. However, stress that overcomes you can be harmful. In one study, rats who were subjected to electrical shocks they could not control developed weakened immune systems. The rats who could control the shocks did not experience impaired resistance. The researchers then theorized that hope is an important part of the disease-resisting process and that despair can actually diminish the ability to fight illness.

4. **Cultivate Friendship.** Warm relationships can be a factor in a healthy immune system. In a study done on dental students, those with close personal relationships secreted many more immunoglobulins (infection-fighting substances) then did students showing anti-social tendencies.

5. **Don't Smoke.** Smoking can decrease vitamin C levels in your body, as well as irritate the respiratory passages. This promotes infection in the dry, cracked tissues. Nicotine produces cadmium to the smoker and non-smoker alike.

6. **Keep Your Home Humidified.** Exceptionally dry air can be as parching to your respiratory system as cigarette smoke. 30 to 40 percent humidity is recommended for a home. If it is less than that you may want to consider purchasing a humidifier. Turning down the heat is also helpful.

7. **Keep Your Hands Clean.** Wash your hands often, as they are the prime mode of travel for germs and viruses.

8.   **Don't Hug Snifflers!** Cold germs can be spread easier in their early stages, so if someone you love has a cold, hold those hugs off for awhile. The germs lose much of their "punch" after a few days.

PARTS OF THE IMMUNE SYSTEM

The human body has specific areas which are associated with the immune system. They involve: the nervous system, the blood, the circulation, the bowels, and the thymus gland.

Nervous System

Recent research has produced evidence that the central nervous system is closely related to the immune system. The nervous system connects the body to the outside world and reacts to the environment. When one system fails to develop normally, the other is affected. Information is constantly being transmitted from the immune system to the brain and vice versa.

For years it has been known that the nervous system controls and coordinates all of the functions of the body, inluding that of the pituitary gland. This gland masters the entire endocrine network. Chiropractors have known this for a long time. They utilize the neuro-immune relationship in the prevention and treatment of disease.

The nervous system regulates the activities of all the other systems in the body and has three main divisions:

1. The central nervous system, which includes the brain and spinal cord.
2. The peripheral nervous system, made up of the nerves that extend out from the spinal cord and the base of the brain to the various parts of the body.
3. The autonomic nervous system, which regulates internal organs.

These areas contain thousands of feet of nerves in the body. Strong nerves depend upon healthy blood and on the food used daily. We need to be aware of our nervous system and not wait until we have problems develop before we feed it properly.

Nervine Herbs

ALFALFA: It is full of nutrients essential for the function of the central nervous system. Alfalfa contains the amino acid tryptophan, which has been proven to be a nerve sedative.

DANDELION: This herb contains choline and linolenic acid. Choline is essential for the health of the myelin sheaths of the nerves.

FENUGREEK: It contains niacin, which helps strengthen the nerves and prevent migraine headaches.

GOTU KOLA: Gotu Kola is rich in B-complex vitamins, which are essential to the maintenance of the nervous system. Feeds and nourishes the brain.

HOPS: Very rich in B vitamins to nourish the nerves. Calming for the nerves, relaxes the body and builds up the nervous system to protect the immune system from damage.

KELP: Kelp is rich in iodine and phosphorus, which are two of many wonderful minerals essential for nerve health. They are also excellent for the thyroid.

LADY'S SLIPPER: This herb acts as a tonic to the central nervous system. It is useful in all stressful situations. Good for emotional and anxiety states. Used to help in nervous pain.

LOBELIA: A wonderful herb with a combination of stimulation and relaxation action. It has healing powers with the ability to remove congestion within the body.

PARSLEY: This herb contains poly-unsaturated and saturated fatty acids, which have a positive influence on the nerves. It is also very high in vitamin A, which builds up the immune system.

PASSION FLOWER: It is a quieting, soothing herb for the central nervous system. It helps restore normal function. It has been used in insomnia, hysteria, and convulsions in children.

SCULLCAP: It will cleanse and rebuild malfunctional areas of the spinal cord. It is very useful in alleviating stress due to emotional conflicts, worry, disturbances of digestion, and circulation. Scullcap is an antispasmodic for tremors, spasms and restlessness. This herb is slow-working but has no side effects and is safe and nourishing. It will aid in strengthening the spinal cord, is a liver cleanser and helps prevent hardening of the arteries. It cleans the veins while it soothes the nerves.

WOOD BETONY: This herb acts as a stimulant for the nerves like black tea, but without any harmful ingredients. It strengthens the immune system and nervous system to protect against diseases.

The Blood

Have you ever stopped to reflect on all of the activities which go on in your body every second without your seeming awareness? We seem to take our bodies for granted until one day when something goes wrong. Our bloodstream is one area of which we must take particular care. It is crucial that we eat properly because it is through a clean blood stream that our immune system is kept in top order.

If a person eats junk food, toxins and poisons will afflict the blood via the colon, which is clogged. The kidneys will try to filter out the impurities, and when they can't handle all of the responsibility, the bloodstream shunts the waste to the lungs, which try to eliminate it in the form of mucus. However, the lungs can only deal with a certain amount of congestion and the blood stream tries one last frantic effort to get rid of the poisons--through the pores of the skin. The skin is the largest eliminating organ there is. Poisons in the blood stream will then manifest themselves as pimples, rashes, and assorted other skin disorders. When toxins are circulating around in the blood stream they poison the cells, diminish immunity to disease, and cause a person to feel sick and rundown. It is extremely important, therefore, to keep our bloodstreams clean with proper foods and herbs. An herbal blood cleanser and Pau d'Arco both clean the blood and strengthen the immune system.

Circulation

The circulatory system is responsible for increasing blood supply to the heart muscles and the entire body. Good circulation is essential to the health of the immune system. However, when a person is under severe stress this circulatory network, and consequently the immunity, will suffer. With heart attacks and strokes claiming thousands of lives each year, we cannot ignore the importance of prevention. Proper diet, stress-management, and exercise are three key elements involved in protecting the heart and ensuring that it does not stop before its time.

10

When a person is tense and uptight, the blood vessels become constricted and the heart is forced to pump wildly in order to circulate the blood adequately. This places an undue burden on the heart and overworks it. In time, it becomes weakened to the point that one day the stress placed on it is too much for it to handle. It then stops...hence, a heart attack.

A stroke can be caused by several factors. One of the most common is blockage in one of the main blood vessels. When circulation is stopped or impeded, oxygen to the brain is diminished. Cells in that particular malnourished area die of "asphyxiation." Sometimes it is in the area of the brain that controls speech, sometimes the area that dictates muscular reflexes.

Clots will often form and obstruct circulation to the brain or heart. Sometimes plaques of cholesterol will adhere and collect on the walls of the blood vessels. Compare this to pipes in a house in which hard water deposits minerals as it flows through them. Over a period of time, the pipes become clogged. When pipes are blocked, plumbing goes haywire. It is the same with our "life-line" pipes, our blood vessels. They are vital links to LIFE. The American Heart Association advises to reduce blood cholesterol by increasing intake of fresh fruits, vegetables and lean meats. It suggests that intake of fatty meats and dairy products be reduced. However, the human body needs a certain amount of cholesterol, and if not supplied through diet, will manufacture its own in the liver or intestine.

Reducing the intake of sugars and other refined carbohydrates, red meat, white flour products, combined with increased activity (such as walking and jumping on a mini-trampoline) will help lower blood fat and cholesterol levels. This will go a long way toward promoting a high caliber immune system.

Circulation is improved with the following nutrients:
Butcher's Broom
Capsicum
Garlic
Gentian Root
Hawthorn Berries
Kelp
Licorice Root
Lecithin
Vitamin E

Bowels

There was a case of a young man who had felt sick for years. It was nothing intense, but just enough to make him feel listless, tired, and depressed. His medical doctors prescribed an assortment of medications but nothing seemed to help. Finally, he went to a chiropractor who was also trained in nutrition.

After a few simple urine tests and an examination of his diet, the doctor diagnosed the young man's problem as "auto-intoxication." His body was literally being poisoned by his intestinal tract.

"Auto-intoxication" or "intestinal toxemia" is a condition brought on by eating the wrong types and amounts of food which certain bacteria will thrive upon, then produce toxins. These toxins then permeate the bloodstream and are carried into the rest of the body. Symptoms of auto-intoxication include fatigue, nervousness, gastrointestinal conditions, skin diseases, headaches, endocrine and circulatory disturbances and others.

The young man was placed on a regime of low-protein, high complex-carbohydrate, low-fat foods, the main emphasis on raw fruits and vegetables. Within one month he felt great. His symptoms gradually disappeared. He states, "It is really frustrating to think that I suffered so long when the answer to my problem was a change in diet. For me, the diet changes weren't that hard. After a while you get so sick of being sick that you're willing to try almost anything. The relief that I feel today has made it worthwhile." The toxins which are formed and sent into the bloodstream are first sent to the liver, which can filter out some, but not all, of them. They are then sent back into the

12

bloodstream to poison various cells. They are finally excreted by the kidneys into the urine and, therefore, their presence can be detected through a urinalysis.

Medical literature has published findings supporting the link between illness and intestinal toxemia:

ALLERGIES: One doctor studies 472 cases; the allergies cleared up when the intestinal toxemia was eliminated.

ASTHMA: Another doctor, after 23 years of observation, stated that toxemia is the underlying cause of the condition and that "the results of treatment justify my position."

ARTHRITIS: Roughly 50% of all cases of inflammatory arthritis can be greatly helped by removing the toxins formed in the intestine."

IRREGULAR HEARTBEATS: About 25% of all cases respond well to elimination of toxemia.

EAR, NOSE AND THROAT DISEASES: "Several hundreds of cases" reported in the scientific literature were from auto-intoxications.

TOXEMIA OF PREGNANCY: In many cases this is from a high protein diet combined with intestinal stagnation (constipation).

EYE DISEASE: Many cases respond well when intestinal toxins are eliminated from the picture.

NERVOUS SYSTEM DISEASES: Both mental and physical diseases may result from auto-intoxication. A paper read at the annual meeting of the American Medical Association in 1917 reported 517 cases of mental symptoms ranging from mental sluggishness to hallucinations that were relieved by eliminating intestinal toxemia. More modern research has related toxemia to schizophrenia.

SENILITY: Even the process of aging may be speeded up by such poisons in the body.

LOW BACK PAIN AND SCIATICA: Sometimes the nerves can be irritated by intestinal toxins and cause these painful conditions.

SKIN DISEASES: One doctor reported a statistical analysis of 900 patients and concluded that "intestinal toxemia is an important causative factor in the production of many skin diseases."

BREAST DISEASE: Many causes of breast pathology have self-healed when the auto-intoxicating process was been alleviated.

CANCER: Sir W.A. Lane, a prominent English surgeon, recorded his feeling of being "exceedingly impressed by the sequence of cancer and intestinal stasis."

The answer to many health problems returns to the same conclusion. Build up the immune system with a healthy diet! Eat a high complex-carbohydrate, low-fat diet with an abundance of fruits and vegetables!

Thymus

One of the most important components of the immune system is the tiniest. Located in your lower neck is the thymus gland, the master gland of the immune system. It is responsible for manufacturing T-cells, white blood cells, commonly known as "T-Lymphocytes." T-cells multiply in order to outnumber the enemy virus. They then migrate throughout the body, keeping a sharp watch for virus-infested cells. They then send a toxin which irritates the offended tissue and draws the "macrophages" or scavenger cells to join the war. Antibodies which are produced by organs having a large number of T-cells adhere to the viruses until the macrophages can devour them.

The thymus manufactures vital hormones involved in the immune process, one of them being "thymosin." The thymus gland will actually shrivel under stress and nutrients, especially vitamin A and zinc, are needed to keep it functioning properly. Vitamin A increases the body's ability to produce "antigens." (An antigen is an enemy substance to which the body reacts by producing antibodies.) Zinc deficiency has been linked to lack of immunity by lowering activity of the T-cells. This, in turn, encourages the growth of infections, neo-plastic and auto-immune diseases.

The mode of travel for lymphocytes throughout the body is lymphatic fluid. Exercise promotes expansion and compression of lymph vessels, thus encouraging the lymphocytes and increasing immune function.

Nutrients play an integral role in building the immune system. Herbs, as well as the vitamins and minerals contained in them are vital to our health. They supply the unique elements which the cells use to strengthen resistance to disease. Below is a list of herbs which are helpful.

14

HERBS TO PROTECT THE IMMUNE SYSTEM

Burdock	Fennel	Plantain
Capsicum	Garlic	Parsley
Catnip	Juniper Berries	Sarsaparilla
Chaparral	Kelp	Shepherd's Purse
Comfrey	Lobelia	Stinging Nettle
Echinacea	Mullein	Watercress

These herbs are called "sulphur herbs." They contain the element sulphur which helps to dissolve acids in the system. It also acts as an antiseptic and strengthens the tissues and blood. Some of these herbs boast an abundance of sulphur and some have only humble amounts.

BURDOCK: Burdock is one of the best blood purifiers. It can reduce swelling around joints and helps rid calcification deposits because it promotes kidney function to help clear the blood of harmful acids. Burdock contains a high amount of vitamin C and iron. It contains 12% protein, 70% carbohydrate, some vitamin A, P, and B-complex, vitamin E, PABA, and small amounts of sulphur, silicon, copper, iodine, and zinc.

CAPSICUM: Capsicum, also known as cayenne, is said to be unequalled for warding off diseases and equalizing blood circulation. It is called a "supreme and harmless internal disinfectant." This herb is a very important one when you want quick action for the flu and colds. Capsicum is high in vitamins A, C, iron and calcium. It has vitamin G, magnesium, phosphorus, and sulphur. It has some B-complex, and is rich in potassium.

CATNIP: Catnip helps in fatigue and improves circulation. It helps in aches and pain, upset stomach and diarrhea associated with flu. Catnip is high in vitamins A and C, and the B-complex. It contains magnesium, manganese, phosphorus, sodium, and has a trace of sulphur.

CHAPARRAL: Chaparral has the ability to cleanse deep into the muscles and tissue walls. It is a potent healer to the urethral tract and lymphatics, tones up the system and rebuilds the tissues. It is one of the best herbal antibiotics. Chaparral has been said to be able to rid the

15

body of LSD residue. Chaparral is high in protein, potassium, and sodium. It also contains silicon, tin, aluminum, sulphur, chlorine, and barium.

COMFREY: Comfrey is one of the most valuable herbs known to botanic medicine. It has a beneficial effect on all parts of the body, being used as an over-all tonic. It is one of the finest healers for the respiratory system, and can be used both internally and externally for healing of fractures, wounds, sores, and ulcers. Comfrey is rich in vitamins A and C. It is high in calcium, potassium, phosphorus, and protein. It contains iron, magnesium, sulphur, copper and zinc, as well as eighteen amino acids.

ECHINACEA: Echinacea stimulates the immune response, increasing the body's ability to resist infections. It improves lymphatic filtration and drainage, and helps remove toxins from the blood. It is considered one of the best blood cleansers and is called the King of the Blood Purifiers. It is considered a non-toxic way of cleansing the system. Echinacea is a natural antibiotic. It contains vitamins A, E and C, iron, iodine, copper, sulphur, and potassium.

FENNEL: Fennel helps stabilize the nervous system and moves waste material out of the body. Fennel improves digestion and has a diuretic effect. It is also helpful in cases of cough and persistent bronchitis, with its mucus-countering and anti-convulsive properties. Fennel contains potassium, sulphur and sodium.

GARLIC: Garlic is nature's antibiotic. It has a rejuvenative effect on all body functions. It is a health building and disease preventive herb and dissolves cholesterol in the bloodstream. Garlic stimulates the lymphatic system to throw off waste materials. It contains antibiotics that are effective against bacteria which may be resistant to other antibiotics. It is called Russian penicillin. Garlic does not destroy the body's normal flora. This herb contains vitamins A and C. It also contains selenium, which is closely related to vitamin E in biological activity. It contains sulphur, calcium, manganese, copper, and a lot of vitamin B1. Garlic also contains some iron and it is high in potassium and zinc.

JUNIPER BERRIES: Juniper is used in cases where uric acid is being retained in the system. It is an excellent disease preventative. It is high in natural insulin. It has the ability to restore the pancreas where there has been no permanent damage. It is excellent for infections.

16

Juniper is high in vitamin C. It contains sulphur, copper, and a high content of cobalt, a trace of tin and aluminum.

KELP: Kelp is a good promoter of glandular health. It has a beneficial effect on many disorders of the body. It is called a sustainer to the nervous system and the brain, helping the brain to function normally. It is essential during pregnancy. Kelp contains nearly 30 minerals. It is rich in iodine, calcium, sulphur and silicon. It is rich in B-complex vitamins.

LOBELIA: Lobelia is a valuable herb. It is well known for removing obstructions from any part of the system. It is very powerful for removing disease and promoting health. It has healing powers with the ability to remove congestion within the body, especially the blood vessels. Lobelia contains sulphur, iron, cobalt, selenium, sodium, copper, and lead.

MULLEIN: Mullein has the ability to loosen mucus and move it out of the body. It is valuable for all lung problems because it nourishes as well as strengthens. The hot tea helps when applied to mumps, tumors, sore throat, and tonsilitis. Mullein is high in iron, magnesium, potassium, and sulphur. It contains vitamins A, D and B-complex.

PLANTAIN: Plantain will neutralize the stomach acids and normalize all stomach secretions. It is known to also neutralize poisons. It clears the ears of mucus. Plantain is rich in vitamins C, K and T. It is rich in calcium, potassium, and sulphur. There is a high content of trace minerals.

PARSLEY: Parsley should be used as a preventative herb. It is so nutritious that it increases resistance to infections and diseases. Parsley is high in vitamin B and potassium. It is said to contain a substance in which cancerous cells cannot multiply. It is rich in iron, chlorophyll, and vitamins A and C. Parsley increases iron content in the blood. It contains some sodium, copper, thiamine and riboflavin. It also has some silicon, sulphur, calcium and cobalt.

SARSAPARILLA: Sarsaparilla is a valuable herb used in glandular balance formulas. It increases circulation to rheumatic joints. It stimulates breathing in congestion problems. Sarsaparilla contains vitamin B-complex, vitamins A, C and D. It also has iron, manganese, sodium, silicon, sulphur, copper, zinc, and iodine.

17

SHEPHERD'S PURSE: Shepherd's Purse is used for cases of hemorrhages after childbirth, excessive menstruation and for internal bleeding of the lungs, colon and hemorrhoids. It acts as a stimulant and moderate tonic for catarrh of the urinary tract indicated by mucus in the urine. Shepherd's Purse is high in vitamin C. It also contains vitamins E and K. It has iron, magnesium, calcium, potassium, tin, zinc, sodium, and sulphur.

STINGING NETTLE: Nettle is one of the most useful of all plants according to folks of the old world in Europe. They have learned this from centuries of experience. It has been said that "the sting of the Nettle is but nothing compared to the pains that it heals." (LeLord Kordels' *Natural Folk Remedies*.) The plant contains alkaloids that neutralize uric acid. It is rich in iron, silicon, and potassium. It is rich in vitamins A and C. It contains a high content of protein. It also contains vitamins E, F and P, calcium, sulphur, sodium, copper, manganese, chromium, and zinc. It also has calcium and vitamin D.

WATERCRESS: Watercress is used principally as a tonic, for regulating the metabolism and the flow of bile. It helps in increasing physical endurance and stamina. Eaten fresh daily, it is a very useful blood purifier and tonic to help supply needed vitamins and minerals. Watercress is an overall excellent food for enriching the blood in anemia and a good remedy in most blood and skin disorders. Experiments have proven that the dried leaves contain three times as much vitamin C as the leaves of lettuce. This plant is very rich in vitamins A, C and D. It is one of the best sources of vitamin E. It also contains vitamins B and G. It is high in iron, iodine, calcium, copper, sulphur and manganese.

One of the most important functions of sulphur-bearing herbs, with their vital minerals, vitamins, and amino acids, is to protect the body from "free radicals," which destroy the immune system. A *free radical* is a toxic chemical which is wildly out of control. It is capable of putting a chemical hole in any tissue of the body. It could destroy a gene or cause a cell wall to leak. When it causes damage to the cell it liberates more free radicals, which in turn damage other cells. In our youth, we produce enzymes that destroy free radicals. However, as we age enzyme production declines, making the body vulnerable. In our modern day existence we come in contact with a myriad of toxic substances daily. These are poisonous agents that can create free

18

radicals. Some of them are pollutants like cigarette smoke, lead, cadmium, sodium nitrite, sulfur dioxide, radiation, and toxic residues from car exhaust. Stress and rancid oil in the diet are also contributing factors of free radicals.

MINERALS FOR THE IMMUNE SYSTEM

CALCIUM: This element is healing to the body. It prevents heavy metals from accumulating in the body. Without adequate calcium the body absorbs heavy metals. It is destroyed by aspirin, coffee, stress, lack of exercise, lack of magnesium, lack of hydrochloric acid, mineral oil and oxalic acid.
CHROMIUM: Although only needed in small amounts by the body, this mineral is critical in fighting foreign bodies.
IODINE: This helps the thyroid gland produce the hormone thyroxine. It also helps the body absorb vitamin A. Lack of this nutrient can cause loss of interest in living and can promote a tendency to get fat.
MAGNESIUM: When a person is deficient in this mineral they can experience a personality change. Magnesium produces properdin, a blood protein that fights invading viruses and bacteria. It is destroyed by alcohol, diuretics, white sugar, white flour, and a high protein diet.
MANGANESE: It activates enzymes that work with vitamin C. As a team, they fight toxins and free radicals. It also stimulates the release of histamine, which protects the immune system. It is destroyed by high meat intake, excess phosphorus, and calcium.
SELENIUM: This is one of the "stars of the show." It is critical and is needed in only small amounts in the body, therefore, is considered a trace mineral. 300 mcg. daily are considered safe for human consumption. It manifests anti-carcinogenic (anti-cancer) and anti-mutagenic (prevents disorders leading to birth defects) properties. Cancer rates are lowest in regions with selenium-rich soil. Selenium inhibits breast, skin, liver, and colon cancer. Selenium is lost in food processing. Brown rice has fifteen times the selenium content of white rice. Whole wheat bread contains twice as much as white bread. Selenium and vitamin E work together to protect the body's cells. It is essential to the body's production of glutathione peroxidase, an enzyme that disarms free radicals.

19

ZINC: This mineral produces histamine, which dilates the capillaries so that blood, carrying immune-fighting white blood cells, can hurry to the scene of an infection.

VITAMINS FOR THE IMMUNE SYSTEM

The following three vitamins are important for many reasons. However, they are most famous for their antioxidant qualities. (An antioxidant helps to protect cells from being robbed of oxygen, which is essential to their functioning. Without adequate oxygen, cells can deteriorate and die. Or it can impair them and make them sick enough to reproduce erratically. This can lead to disorders like cancer. Free radicals smother cells so that oxygen cannot be properly utilized.)

VITAMIN A: Vitamin A increases resistance to infections. Deficiencies increase chances of viral, bacterial and protozoal invasions, and their severity. It is an essential nutrient to protect against cancer. Laboratory evidence shows that vitamin A is able to suppress chemically induced tumors. This vitamin is involved with the maintenance of epithelial linings and mucous membranes, which are the first places that are penetrated by invaders. Vitamin A protects against the effects of all types of pollution. The protection of vitamin A seems to be most evident among smokers. It reduces susceptibility to respiratory problems, i.e., colds, sinusitis, asthma, bronchitis, ear infections, and cystic fibrosis. It increases immunity against environmental pollution such as pesticides and herbicides. It works with zinc for optimum efficiency. Vitamin A is destroyed by high heat.

VITAMIN E: This vitamin prevents the oxidized state that cancer cells thrive in. It deactivates the free radicals that promote cellular damage leading to malignancy. Deficiencies of vitamin E depress general resistance to disease. Its blood thinning properties help dissolve blood clots and keep the arteries from clogging. The anti-oxidant characteristics are useful in retarding the aging process. Bacteria, viruses, and cancer cells respond to larger amounts of vitamin E than recommended in RDA. Processing and storage of food destroys some of the vitamin E content of most foods.

VITAMIN C: This vitamin plays a role in the formation of connective tissue in the body. It also helps the body's absorption of iron. More

20

importantly, however, vitamin C has shown even more powerful effects through animal, human and test-tube studies. They've demonstrated that this vitamin can activate white blood cells to battle foreign substances and increase the production of interferon, the body's anti-virus protein. Vitamin C also has a talent for killing disease-inducing bacteria. Vitamin C can be affected by exposure to light, long-term storage of foods, heat and canning.

Essential Fatty Acids

EVENING PRIMROSE OIL: Evening Primrose Oil contains high amounts of PGE, a vitamin-like compound involved in proper function of the immune system. A shortage of PGE is believed to cause abnormal and harmful immune response. It stimulates the T-cells of the immune system. Experiments done in test tubes show that it reverts cancer cells back to normal cells. PGE is required for the T-cells of the immune system to attack cancer. T-cells are the main mechanism of the immune system to protect the body from foreign cells, viruses, bacteria, fungi, and allergens.

B Vitamins

B vitamins protect the immune and nervous systems. They help build blood, protect the body against infection and help produce antibodies. They increase production of hydrochloric acid for digestion, and are very vital in helping stablize mood swings. These are the vitamins that support the immune system by reducing the impact of stress in one's life.

B-1 (THIAMINE): This B-complex vitamin is helpful for cell respiration, metabolism of carbohydrates, a healthy heart and proper growth of the body.

B-2 (RIBOFLAVIN): It is used by the body to metabolize proteins and lipids, supplies oxygen to the cells and is used by the skin and nails. It is especially needed during stressful situations.

B-3 (NIACIN): This nutrient stimulates circulation. It aids memory function, releases histamines and helps in hyperactivity. It is an excellent vitamin for the nerves. It is essential for brain metabolism. It reduces tension, fatigue, depression and insomnia.

21

B-5 (PANTOTHENIC ACID): It protects against respiratory infections and is a natural tranquilizer.

B-6 (PYRIDOXINE): The body uses B-6 in hormone and antibody production, in the synthesis of DNA and RNA and in the metabolism of fat, protein and carbohydrates. It is nature's diuretic and is very useful in menstruation and the water gained at this time. It is excellent for insomnia.

B-12: This nutrient increases the body's resistance to infection. A person especially needs this vitamin when fatigued. It helps form red blood cells, and helps prevent constipation.

BIOTIN: It is used for the proper functioning of skin, nerves, bone marrow, and reproductive glands. It helps metabolize carbohydrates and protein.

CHOLINE: This helps keep the nerve coverings (myelin) healthy, aids in production of acetycholine (a neurotransmitter), and helps the body utilize fat and cholesterol.

FOLIC ACID: It is used for red blood cell formation and the synthesis of DNA and RNA.

INOSITOL: Works with choline and is vital for nourishment of the brain. It has been shown to help reduce fat in the liver.

PABA (PARA-AMINOBENZOIC ACID): This vitamin protects the body against free radicals and is part of the folic acid molecule.

According to Arnold Fox, M.D. (Let's Live Magazine, February 1984), the following chart associates his findings of decreased states of the immune system to the following B-complex vitamins:

SEVERE - B-5 (Pantothenic Acid), B-6 (Pyridoxine), and Folic Acid.

MODERATE - B-1 (Thiamine), B-2 (Riboflavin), B-3 (Niacin), and Biotin.

MILD - B-12.

AMINO ACIDS

Sulphur-bearing amino acids are important constituents of the immune system framework. Through the sulphur they are able to make the mineral selenium available to the cells. We know that selenium is helpful in preventing cancer, and pulling heavy metals such as lead, mercury and cadmium from the body. They neutralize and eliminate potentially destructive free radicals which helps in cell immunity. The

22

amino acids methionine, cysteine and taurine work as a team. During dieting methinonine and cysteine will insure adequate taurine to protect the heart muscle from calcium and potassium loss.

METHIONINE: This amino acid helps keep hair, skin, nails and joints healthy. It functions to remove toxic wastes from the liver. Bottle-fed babies frequently have high ammonia content in their urine, which causes ammonia rashes and blisters. Methionine is the antidote.

CYSTEINE: This one is a powerful aid in protecting the body against radiation and pollution. It acts as an antioxidant, destroys free radicals and neutralizes toxins. It can block the chemicals in polluted air and tobacco smoke. Cysteine can negate the effects of acetaldehyde, a dangerous irritant. This toxic material is found in smog and cigarette smoke. It helps stop the toxic metals, mercury and cadmium from damaging sensitive tissue. It's antioxidant properties are enhanced when combined with vitamin E.

TAURINE: This is not an essential amino acid for most adults but is for infants. Mother's milk contains plenty of taurine, but cow's milk doesn't. It is critical in brain development. This amino acid is concentrated in the heart, skeletal, muscle and central nervous system. It has a potent and long-lasting anti-convulsive effect. It helps to normalize the balance of other amino acids, which in epilepsy are thoroughly disordered. Taurine is associated with zinc in healthy eye function. It protects the loss of potassium in the heart muscle. It's synthesis in humans is derived from the amino acids methionine and cysteine.

The following are more amino acids which play a vital role in aiding the immune system:

TRYPTOPHAN: This acid cleanses toxins from the blood stream.

GLYCINE: It helps in building antibody action.

L-CYSTEINE: This one combats free radicals and promotes healing of wounds.

GLUTAMIC ACID: This nutrient is vital in proper brain function.

L-LYSINE: This is one of the eight essential amino acids that the body must obtain from an outside source. It may lessen the incidence of some kinds of cancer. This amino acid can change one enzyme. It would appear that a single amino acid shift may underlie malignancy.

FOOD SOURCES OF IMMUNE BUILDERS

Minerals

CALCIUM: Milk and milk products, all cheeses, soybeans, sardines, salmon, peanuts, walnuts, sunflower seeds, dried beans, green vegetables.
CHROMIUM: Meat, shellfish, chicken, corn oil, clams, brewer's yeast.
IODINE: Kelp, vegetables grown in iodine-rich soil, onions, and all seafood.
MAGNESIUM: Figs, lemons, grapefruit, yellow corn, almonds, nuts, seeds, dark green vegetables, apples.
MANGANESE: Nuts, green leafy vegetables, peas, beets, egg yolks, whole wheat cereals.
SELENIUM: Wheat germ, bran, tuna, onions, tomatoes, broccoli.
ZINC: Round steak, lamb chops, pork loin, wheat germ, brewer's yeast, pumpkin seeds, eggs, nonfat dry milk, ground mustard.

Vitamins

VITAMIN A: Orange and bright green fruits and vegetables, peppers, peaches, apricots, cod liver oil, carrots, yams.
VITAMIN E: Wheat germ, nuts, sweet potatoes, corn, sunflower oil, spinach, watercress, tomatoes.
VITAMIN C: Most fruits and vegetables, especially citrus fruits and green peppers.

B-Complex Vitamins

B-1 (THIAMINE): Whole grain wheat, whole grain oats, lentils, navy beans, pinto beans, red beans, and many vegetables.
B-2 (RIBOFLAVIN): Mushrooms, millet, split peas, barley, parsley, broccoli, chicken, turkey, lentils, many beans, okra, almonds.
B-3 (NIACIN): Turkey, chicken, brown rice, buckwheat, mushrooms, barley, red chili peppers, split peas, dates, and brewer's yeast.
B-5 (PANTOTHENIC ACID): Foods include whole grains, green vegetables, nuts, meats and fish.

B-6 (PYRIDOXINE): Cantaloupe, tuna, lentils, buckwheat, whole grain rice, bananas, whole grain rye, spinach, potatoes, and many other fruits and vegetables.

B-12: Liver, milk, eggs, meat, cheese, miso, and soy sauce.

BIOTIN: Peas, peanuts, beans, lentils, milk, whole grain rice, beef liver, fish, and other whole grains.

CHOLINE: Lecithin, leafy green vegetables, oats, soybeans, egg yolks, and liver.

FOLIC ACID: Fresh dark green vegetables, carrots, cantaloupes, apricots, beans, whole wheat flour, endive, asparagus and turnips.

INOSITOL: Cabbage, grapefruit, cantaloupe, peanuts, raisins, lima beans, and brewer's yeast.

Sulphur Amino Acids

These are found in eggs, dried peas, and beans and garlic.

EXERCISE

If you exercise even as little as fifteen minutes a day, the germ-fighting white blood cells of your body will be increased. To be effective, you must raise your resting pulse 50% and keep it raised for fifteen minutes. The lymphatic system responds to the stimulation of exercise when using the rebounder (mini-trampoline). It is best if you use it for short periods several times per day. As a result of this daily program, deeper breathing and exhaling will come naturally. This will increase oxygen in the blood and brain. It will also increase the circulation of blood and lymphatic fluid, thus protecting the immune system. Exercise helps minimize stress and its detrimental effects on the body. Mark Bricklin, in *The Practical Encyclopedia of Natural Healing* (Rodale Press), states: "Exercise is basic to health. It burns up cholesterol and other fats. It improves circulation to the point that areas which are stressed with regular exercise will actually develop additional tiny blood vessels to deliver oxygen and remove wastes. Muscles trained by exercise develop greater stores of ready energy in the form of glycogen. The muscles themselves grow larger and stronger. Lung function improves and the heart rate becomes lower. The secret, I believe, to the effective use of exercise as a therapy is to develop an avid interest not so much in exercise itself, but in some hobby which requires vigorous movements of all kinds. Some of the best are swimming, folk dancing, yoga, Tai-Chai, karate, tennis, gardening and hiking."

POSITIVE MENTAL ATTITUDE

The famous P.M.A. master, Napoleon Hill, says, "Kil! the habit of worry, in all its forms, by reaching a general, blanket decision that nothing which life has to offer is worth the price of worry. With this decision will come poise, peace of mind, and calmness of thought which will bring happiness.

Your business in life is, presumably, to achieve success. To be successful, you must find peace of mind, acquire material needs of life, and above all, attain happiness. All of these evidences of success begin in the form of thought impulses. You may control your own mind, you have the power to feed it whatever thought impulses you choose. With this privilege goes also the responsibility of using it constructively." Many studies and much research has been conducted which proves that a positive state of mind boosts the body's immunity by releasing infection-fighting T-cells from the thymus gland.

DESTROYERS OF THE IMMUNE SYSTEM

There are many "immune system destroyers." We are bombarded daily with them and they come in many forms, sometimes even disguises. We will cover some of the most common ones. How many do you recognize as part of *your* life?

AGENE (Nitrogen Trichloride): This is used to bleach flour and give it a snowy white appearance. However, it can cause epileptic-like fits and ataxia (failure of muscle coordination).

ALCOHOL: Excessive use of alcohol creates a severely impaired immune system. It increases susceptibility to infection. It weakens the central nervous system. It promotes chronic lung disease, malignancies of the neck and head, intestinal problems, hypoglycemia, diabetes, liver disease and many other problems. Alcohol depletes B

26

vitamins, folic acid, niacin, Vitamin E, magnesium, zinc, and protein. All of the nutrients that alcohol depletes play a critical role in immune health.

ASPARTAME (Equal, NutraSweet): Aspartame breaks down in the digestive tract as a toxic material called "methanol." To prevent methanol from metabolizing into the poison formaldehyde, a person needs to take another poison, ethanol (alcohol).

GLUTAMIC ACID: This substance is found in the flavor enhancer, monosodium glutamate. It affects the central nervous system and can trigger depression, gloomy fantasies and rage as long as two weeks after eating foods with M.S.G.

HIGH-FAT DIET: A high fat intake increases levels of bile acids in the colon. This breaks down into deoxycholic and lithocholic acids, which are cancer-causing elements. This can cause cancer of the colon and rectum. Cancer of the pancreas, breast, gallbladder, ovaries, uterus, prostate, and leukemia are correlated with a diet high in animal protein and fat. High-fat diets and obesity also are linked with the incidence of breast cancer.

JUNK FOOD (Sweets, White Flour, White Sugar Products): These put a double stress on the body. When too much junk food is eaten, the appetite for wholesome food is dulled.

CAFFEINE: Caffeine decreases immunity. Fibrocystic breast disease is connected with the consumption of foods containing caffeine. It is caused by the chemicals methylxanthine, theophylline, and theobromine, which are found in coffee, black tea, cola drinks, chocolate, and other soft drinks. These elements act on hormones that cause breast tissue to develop fibrocystic lumps. Caffeine robs the body of its use of iron and inositol, and is a suspect in causing cancer of the pancreas.

FOOD DYES, FLAVORINGS: These culprits have been indicted as potent factors in behavioral problems in children and adults. Some of these problems are learning disabilities and hyperkinesis (hyperactivity).

SODIUM NITRITE: It is a preservative found in cured meats like hot dogs, bologna, ham, etc. It is capable of producing seemingly permanent epileptic changes in brain activity and damage to the central nervous system.

MEAT: High protein diets can deplete calcium in the body. This is especially true if the source is an animal product. In beef there are

27

concentrated doses of hormones and antibiotics. These suppress the immune system and promote tumor growths.

POLY-UNSATURATED FATS: Fats undergo a process called lipid peroxidation, which produces rancidity in oils. This process releases dangerous free radicals. It is suspected that the increase of poly-unsaturated fats in the diet is the cause of high cancer rates in the United States.

HEAVY METALS: Food, water and air are contaminated with lead, cadmium, and mercury. Even small amounts are considered toxic. They cause serious damage to the nervous system. They are also implicated in learning disabilities and behavioral disorders.

1. Cadmium--Cadmium, found in cigarette smoke, is harmful to non-smokers as well as smokers. Cadmium levels depress bone marrow function and antibody response. Cadmium is an industrial, environmental pollutant. It competes with zinc in the body and a high zinc level will help eliminate cadmium.

2. Lead--Lead weakens the immune system. It is found in auto exhaust, smog, some white paints. It can contaminate food and water. It causes brain damage, neuritis, and kidney cancer.

3. Mercury--This poison is found in shellfish. Small ocean fish are usually safe. The mercury component of the amalgam used in dental fillings is toxic. Mercury can cause lymphoid tissue changes and depresses vital cells that battle in the immune system.

VACCINATIONS AND ANTIBIOTICS: The wide spread use of vaccinations and antibiotics is considered one of the main causes of immune system disorders.

Dr. Robert Mendelsohn says, "There is a growing suspicion that immunization against relatively harmless childhood diseases may be responsible for the dramatic increase in autoimmune diseases since mass inoculations were introduced."

Autoimmune diseases, such as AIDS, Alzheimer's, asthma, allergies, cancer, lupus, and multiple sclerosis, to name a few, are the epidemic plagues of our times. A large part of the population of the United States suffers from one or more of these disorders chronically. As long as we play games with the immune system and interfere with the body's only protection we will see more and more unusual autoimmune diseases that we never would have dreamed possible.

28

STRESS

Stressful situations leach out nutrients from our body at an astonishing rate. The B-complex vitamins are especially deficient in the American diet and the body's resistance drops very low when they are lacking. Folic acid and vitamin B-12 are involved in the maintenance of the immune system and therefore, help in the inhibition of aging. Low levels of essential vitamins and minerals reduce the tolerance to stress. Stress, in a sense, is toxic because it causes free radicals to form in the body. Herbs can help relax the body, without side effects. One herb to relieve the effects of stress is Passion Flower. It is a natural tranquilizer and will relax tension in the nervous system. It helps to control high blood pressure. It is great for exhaustion. It tones the nerve centers, improves the circulation and gives nutrition to feed the nerves. It will take the place of narcotics without the side effects and will not destroy the nerves like drugs do. It contains *passiflorine*, which is similar in effect to morphine.

Stress and Depression

Stress, depression and prolonged grief have an effect on the physical/chemical response of the immune system. Depressed persons suffer more illness than the happy person. Depression causes less T- and B-cells to respond. It also diminishes lymphocyte production in the body. Severe emotional stress can cause shrinkage of the thymus gland. Even a person's thoughts have a definite effect on the immune system. The mind is a powerful instrument and can convince the body it is ill. It is possible to think you have ulcers. The stress the mind puts on the body actually can induce ulcers! The body responds to negative emotions, but also responds to positive ones.

Relax and Daydream

A wonderful way to relax and escape from pressures is to daydream. Find a quiet, peaceful place to think...a day in the mountains, beach or park. Think beautiful, peaceful thoughts...listen to the birds, trees, wind...smell the fresh air...walk barefoot in the grass...feel the sun warming your body.

Replace all your fears and stress with loving, positive thoughts--memories of loved ones. Do you experience panic attacks? These are feelings of being unable to cope and being frightened. If you ever experience this, take a deep breath, let it slowly out. Take another deep big breath, and continue. Tips for alleviating worry, stress, and depression are:

1. Write your worries down.
2. Get away for awhile.
3. Release tension by crying.
4. Exercise out aggression.
5. Laugh and smile...don't take yourself too seriously.
6. Always endeavor to learn new things.
7. Realize your worth.

The Mind and Stress

The mind reacts to stress in tightening of muscles, impairment of blood flow to organs, constriction of the lungs, irregular heartbeat, high blood pressure, or changes of the immune system. Those people most susceptible to these symptoms are those who are always in a hurry, quick to anger, and always thinking of themselves. How we react to stress is the key. Hypertension is one of the characteristic diseases of our age. One who lives in a fast-paced society is a potential victim of high blood pressure. It is very interesting to observe that an increase in blood pressure is one of the body's normal reactions to fear. It is the body's way of preparing to meet the danger at hand. A temporary increase in blood pressure enables the body to fight or flee--to take whatever action is necessary to overcome the danger. It could be said that the person with high blood pressure lives in a constant state of fear. Unfortunately, this chronic state of readiness for danger is very wearing on the body's system.

Constant stress will cause the weakest part of the body to suffer first. It could cause insomnia, asthma, anxiety, constipation, cancer, ulcers or headaches, to name a few.

Meditation

During this exercise the breathing slows, the blood pressure falls, the pulse slows, and the metabolic rate is lowered. When the mind changes, the body reflects the mind. Thoughts in the mind and pondered cause an effect in the body. It has been found that lactic acid and carbon dioxide do not accumulate in the body when one is meditating. Scientific research reveals that using meditation is more restful to the body than sleep. This is because when we sleep we often tense our muscles and grind our teeth. Using meditation just 15 minutes a day would produce more positive restful feelings than a nap. It will help you gain more control over the immune, circulatory, and cardiovascular systems. Sleep will be more efficient and you will need less of it. You will experience an increased amount of alert, productive hours.

MENUS AND RECIPES

Food can taste delicious as well as be a weapon against disease. For example, broccoli, brussels sprouts and cabbage contain *indoles*, substances which increase chemical reactions in the body to prevent cancerous tumors. Studies show that people who consume more of these foods are less prone to colon and rectal cancer. Chlorophyll in green, leafy vegetables helps reduce cancer-causing agents in the body. Beta-carotene, which gives the yellowish color to fruit and vegetables, is a potent cancer-inhibitor. This substance converts to vitamin A in the liver. It is also found in green vegetables, but the chlorophyll masks the carotene color. The liver stores vitamin A and when stress or disease strike and increase the need for vitamin A, the liver will release enough stored vitamin A to keep the blood levels up. Beta-carotene is valuable because your body will only convert as much as it needs and there is no fear of "overdose." Beta-carotene offers protection against certain cancers, especially cancer of the esophagus, stomach, small intestine, large intestine, rectum, lungs, and skin.

Essential fatty acids in the diet play a vital role, too. They promote T-lymphocyte activity and are indispensible for immune system health. These substances are found in avocadoes, sunflower seeds, nuts, cold water fish, liver and evening primrose oil. Some foods to avoid include: cottonseed oil, some edible mushrooms, burned or browned foods such as charcoaled or flame-broiled meats.

A well-balanced diet consists of fresh fruits and vegetables, nuts, seeds, beans, and whole grains. YOU ARE WHAT YOU EAT!

The following are considered anti-stress foods.

Chicken	Brussels Sprouts	Prunes
Turkey	Cherries	Plums
Fish	Corn	Tomatoes
Apples	Leaf Lettuce (green)	Watercress
Apricots	Melons	Brown Rice
Bananas	Okra	Pineapple
Green & Wax Beans	Parsley	Yellow Cornmeal
Berries	Peaches	Rye
Broccoli	Fresh Peas	Millet
Cabbage	Potatoes	Goat's Milk

The Federal Government has initiated cancer prevention research...to begin looking toward PREVENTION rather than CURE. LET'S LOOK TO THE KITCHEN, RATHER THAN THE RESEARCH LABS!

SEVEN-DAY SUGGESTED MENU

In most cases vitamins, minerals and herbs are best taken with meals. If digestion is a problem, digestive enzymes and hydrochloric acid can be added. Fresh fruit and vegetables and juices can be eaten between meals. Herbal teas help protect the immune system: Red Clover, Alfalfa, Pau d'Arco, Red Raspberry, and Licorice.

The following recipes are taken from *Today's Healthy Eating* by Louise Tenney. The recipes marked with an * are included in this booklet.

#1 Breakfast:
    *Raw Oats with Fruit

32

#1 Lunch:
    *Stuffed Pepper (raw)
    *Almond-Sunflower Seed Muffins

#1 Supper:
    *Pinto Bean Stew
    *Cornbread

#2 Breakfast:
    Fresh Fruit--apple, peach or avocado
    1 C. cooked Millet with Maple Syrup and chopped Almonds,
        with Almond Milk

#2 Lunch:
    *Seed and Vegetable Salad

#2 Supper:
    *Garbanzo Stew
    Fresh Carrot and Celery sticks

#3 Breakfast:
    Fresh Fruit--grapes, banana or apricots
    *Buckwheat Groats

#3 Lunch:
    *Potato Salad with Dressing

#3 Supper:
    *Rice and Nut Casserole
    Fresh Tomatoes with olive oil, garlic and oregano

#4 Breakfast:
    *Mixed Fruit Compote
    10 Almonds

#4 Lunch:
    *Potato Supreme
    Vegetable Salad

#4 Supper:
   *Barley Nut Casserole
   Celery Salad

#5 Breakfast:
   *Yogurt and Fruit

#5 Lunch:
   *Alfalfa and Artichoke Salad

#5 Supper:
   *Lima Bean Roast
   Broccoli, lightly steamed and sautéed in olive oil and
      garlic

#6 Breakfast:
   *Granola
   Almond Milk

#6 Lunch:
   *Lima Bean Salad

#6 Supper:
   *Baked Rice and Millet
   Fresh Vegetable Salad

#7 Breakfast:
   *Whole Wheat Berries
   Nut Milk

#7 Lunch:
   *Raw Soup

#7 Supper:
   *Cheese Enchiladas
   Fresh Vegetable Salad

RECIPES

Breakfast

RAW OATS WITH FRUIT MUESLI

2 T. baby oats	1 T. ground almonds
6 T. spring water	1 T. ground sunflower seeds
2 T. lemon juice	2-3 T. almond milk
1/4 grated fresh apple	1 tsp. maple syrup

Soak oats overnight in spring water. Add lemon juice and almond milk until smooth. Add grated, unpeeled apple. Sprinkle nuts and seeds; add more almond milk if needed.

This recipe can be used with any fresh fruit in season, such as strawberries, raspberries, blueberries, apples, bananas, peaches, apricots. Yogurt can also be added for variety.

BUCKWHEAT GROATS

2 C. buckwheat groats	1 tsp. vegetable salt
2 eggs, lightly beaten	4 C. pure water, boiled

Cook groats and eggs in a heavy skillet over a high heat for a few minutes. Stir constantly to keep eggs from sticking. Add boiling water and reduce heat and simmer, covered, for about 30 minutes. Add vegetable salt before serving.

MIXED FRUIT COMPOTE

2 apples
1 C. dried fruit (apricots,
      white figs, prunes)
1/3 C. currants
1/2 stick cinnamon

Thin lemon slice
1/4 C. almonds, ground
1/2 lemon, juiced
2-1/2 C. water

Slice apples in chunks and put in saucepan with all other ingredients except currants. Brink to boil, then simmer on low heat, covered, for about 30 minutes. Remove the cinnamon stick and lemon slice. Stir in currants and serve for breakfast. Makes about 4 servings.

YOGURT AND FRUIT

2 C. yogurt
2 C. frozen or fresh
      blueberries or
      strawberries
2 ripe bananas, sliced

1 apple, grated
Pure maple syrup
1/2 C. almonds, ground

Fold fruit into yogurt, sweeten with maple syrup to taste. Garnish with ground almonds.

GRANOLA

5 C. rolled oats
3 C. rolled wheat
2 C. wheat germ
1 C. rice polishing
1 C. almonds
1 C. pecans
1 C. walnuts

2 C. sunflower seeds
1 C. bran
2 C. coconut, unsweetned
1 C. flaxseeds, ground
1 C. sesame seeds
1/2 C. chia seeds, ground

Mix dry ingredients together.

1-1/4 C. honey	*1 T. vanilla, pure*
1/4 C. maple syrup	*1 C. raw oil mixed with...*
1/2 C. date sugar	*1 C. hot water*

Mix thoroughly all other ingredients. Spread out in a shallow baking pan. Bake at 325°F. for about 30 minutes or until dry and golden brown, stirring often to prevent burning.

WHEAT BERRIES

1 C. whole wheat	*1/2 tsp. sesame kelp salt*
3 C. spring water	*or sea salt*

Rinse grain. Add slowly to boiling water and add salt. Stir grain with a fork and place lid on pan and reduce heat and simmer for one hour.

It makes a good breakfast food by adding milk or nut milk and a little pure maple syrup.

It can be used in casseroles and ground and used in breads or added to other grain for main dishes or added to cookies for a crunchy taste.

Lunch

STUFFED PEPPERS

2 large green peppers	*3 green onions, chopped*
cut in half	*1 C. peas, fresh or frozen*
1/2 C. celery, chopped	*2 hard cooked egg yolks*
1 C. watercress, chopped	*Homemade mayonnaise to*
1 tomato, chopped	*moisten*

Prepare green peppers and chill in cold water for a few hours. Mix all other ingredients together and fill the green pepper halves just before ready to eat.

ALMOND-SUNFLOWER SEED MUFFINS

1 C. ground sunflower
    seeds
1 C. ground almonds
1/4 C. ground sesame seeds

1/2 C. wheat germ
1/2 C. rice polishings
1/2 C. unsweetened coconut

Combine dry ingredients. Add the following ingredients but fold in egg whites last.

3 egg yolks
2 T. honey
2-1/2 T. cold pressed oil

1 C. orange juice
3 beaten egg whites

Fill greased muffin tins 3/4 full and bake at 350°F. for about 25 minutes.

SEED AND VEGETABLE SALAD

3 C. leaf lettuce
1 C. watercress
1 C, alfalfa sprouts
1/2 C. grated carrots
1/2 C. grated raw beets
1/2 C. red cabbage
1/2 C. chopped celery

2 medium tomatoes, chopped
1 corn on the cob, cut off
1/4 C. fresh peas or frozen
1/2 C. sunflower seeds
1/4 C. sesame seeds
1/4 C. pine nuts
Handful parsley

POTATO SALAD

6 medium potatoes,
    boiled
1 C. grated carrots

1 C. cooked green beans
1 small red onion, chopped
1 C. chopped celery

Dice potatoes with skins on, cut raw carrots in small pieces. Cut cooked green beans lengthwise.

Dressing:

1 clove garlic, crushed
1-1/2 T. vegetable oil
1 T. lemon juice
1 T. thyme
1 C. chopped fresh
    mushrooms

1 T. chopped chives
1/2 C. plain yogurt
1/4 C. buttermilk
2 T. mayonnaise
1 T. prepared mustard
Kelp to taste

Sauté garlic in oil. Add mushrooms. Add lemon juice and thyme.

Combine all other ingredients. Cool sautéed mixture. Mix all together and serve over potato salad.

POTATO SUPREME

Bake 1 potato for each person.

In a saucepan sauté 2 cups mushrooms in 4 tablespoons butter with one clove minced garlic. Simmer lightly; do not let mushrooms get soggy.

Open up potatoes; put in butter, grated cheese, sour cream, chopped black olives and chopped chives. Top with sautéed mushrooms. Use your imagination for baked potatoes (chili, stroganoff, etc.).

ALFALFA AND ARTICHOKE SALAD

2 C. alfalfa sprouts
1 C. Jerusalem artichokes,
    sliced
1 C. tomatoes, sliced
    lengthwise

1 small avocado, diced
1 small green pepper, diced
1 C. carrots, grated
1 C. celery, chopped

LIMA BEAN SALAD

2 C. cooked lima beans
4 hard boiled eggs,
   mashed
1 C. chopped celery
1/2 tsp. chili powder

1/4 C. chopped green
   pepper
4 tsp. chopped onions
1/2 C. homemade
   mayonnaise

Add all ingredients together and mix well. Chill before serving.

RAW SOUP

Raw soups contain live enzymes that are essential to help prevent cancer and other diseases.

3 C. vegetable broth
1 C. tomato juice
1 T. ground chia seeds
   (optional)

1 T. olive oil
1/2 tsp. kelp
2 T. vegetable broth powder

Heat all ingredients and simmer for 10 minutes. Remove from heat and add the following raw vegetables:

1/2 C. grated carrots
1/2 C. grated celery
1/2 C. fresh sweet corn
1/2 C. fresh peas

1 small chopped onion
2 fresh tomatoes, cut in
   small pieces
2 sprigs parsley, chopped

PINTO BEAN STEW

2 C. pinto beans, cooked
4 C. vegetable broth
1 C. carrots, sliced
1/2 C. broccoli, sliced
1/2 C. zucchini
1/2 C. celery, sliced
3 large tomatoes, peeled
and chopped

1/4 C. clarified butter or
olive oil
1/4 C. millet
1/4 C. brown rice
1 T. vegetable seasoning
1 T. kelp

Sauté onions and garlic in butter or oil in a large stew pan. Add all ingredients and water if needed. Bring to a boil, reduce heat and simmer about 45 minutes until rice and millet are cooked.

CORNBREAD

1 C. corn meal
1/2 C. whole wheat flour
1/2 tsp. baking powder
(aluminum free)
1/4 C. wheat germ
2 T. cold pressed oil

1/4 tsp. sea salt
1 egg
1/4 C. honey
1/2 C. yogurt

Mix oil, egg, honey and yogurt. Add salt and baking powder. Stir in flour and corn meal slowly. Butter an 8 x 10-inch glass baking dish. Bake at 400°F. for about 30 minutes until golden brown.

GARBANZO STEW

1 qt. Tomato Supreme or
    tomatoes
1 qt. pure water
1 C. garbanzo beans
1 C. carrots

1 C. potatoes, skins on
1/4 C. millet
1 tsp. mineral salt
1 T. vegetable powder

Soak garbanzo beans overnight in 2 cups water. Cook beans in 1 quart Tomato Supreme or tomatoes (canned), and one quart of water. Cook until tender. Add millet and cook 30 minutes. Add chopped carrots, diced potatoes, salt and vegetable powder.

RICE AND NUT CASSEROLE

2-1/2 C. vegetable stock
1 C. brown rice
1/4 C. ground sesame
    seeds
1/2 C. fresh corn

1 C. chopped tomatoes
2 T. sweet basil
1/2 C. chopped almonds
4 chopped green onions

Sauté onions in 1 tablespoon olive oil; add stock and bring to boil. Stir rice slowly. Reduce heat and simmer for about 45 minutes. Add corn, sesame seeds, tomatoes, basil and almonds. Simmer for about 15 minutes more.

BARLEY NUT CASSEROLE

1 C. barley
1/2 C. chopped almonds
1/2 C. fresh mushrooms
2 T. chopped parsley
2 C. vegetable broth

1/2 C. green onions
2 T. butter
1 T. miso (soybean paste)
1 T. apricot kernels, ground

Sauté mushrooms and onions gently. Place in casserole with all other ingredients. Bake in oven, covered, for 45 minutes at 350°F. (or until barley is tender). Serve with a fresh vegetable salad.

LIMA BEAN ROAST

2 C. lima beans, cooked
1 C. walnuts, ground
3 green onions

1 C. ripe tomatoes
2 T. olive oil
1 tsp. kelp or mineral salt

Blend all together in blender and place in buttered loaf pan. Bake at 350°F. for 45 minutes. Baste with lemon juice and unsalted butter.

BAKED RICE AND MILLET

1-1/2 C. cooked brown
     rice
1/2 C. cooked millet
2 eggs, beaten
2 C. milk

2 T. butter
1 T. tamari soy sauce
1 C. chopped almonds
1/4 C. chopped sunflower
     seeds

Mix all ingredients. Pour into 1-1/2 quart casserole dish. Bake 30 minutes at 350°F.

CHEESE ENCHILADAS

12 corn tortillas
2 C. mild cheese, grated
1/2 C. onions
1 small can diced green
     chiles
1 tall can enchilada sauce

1 small can tomato sauce
1 pint sour cream or mock
     sour cream
Black olives (optional), to
     sprinkle on top

Heat enchilada sauce and tomato sauce and add 1 small can of water. Mix the cheese, onions and chiles. Dip tortilla in the hot sauce mix to soften. Place about 2 T. of the cheese mixture on tortilla, top with a heaping tablespoon of sour cream; roll the tortilla and place seam side down and put in a baking dish. When all the tortillas are rolled up pour the rest of the enchilada sauce on the top and sprinkle top with cheese and olives. Bake in 350°F. oven for about 30 minutes.

43